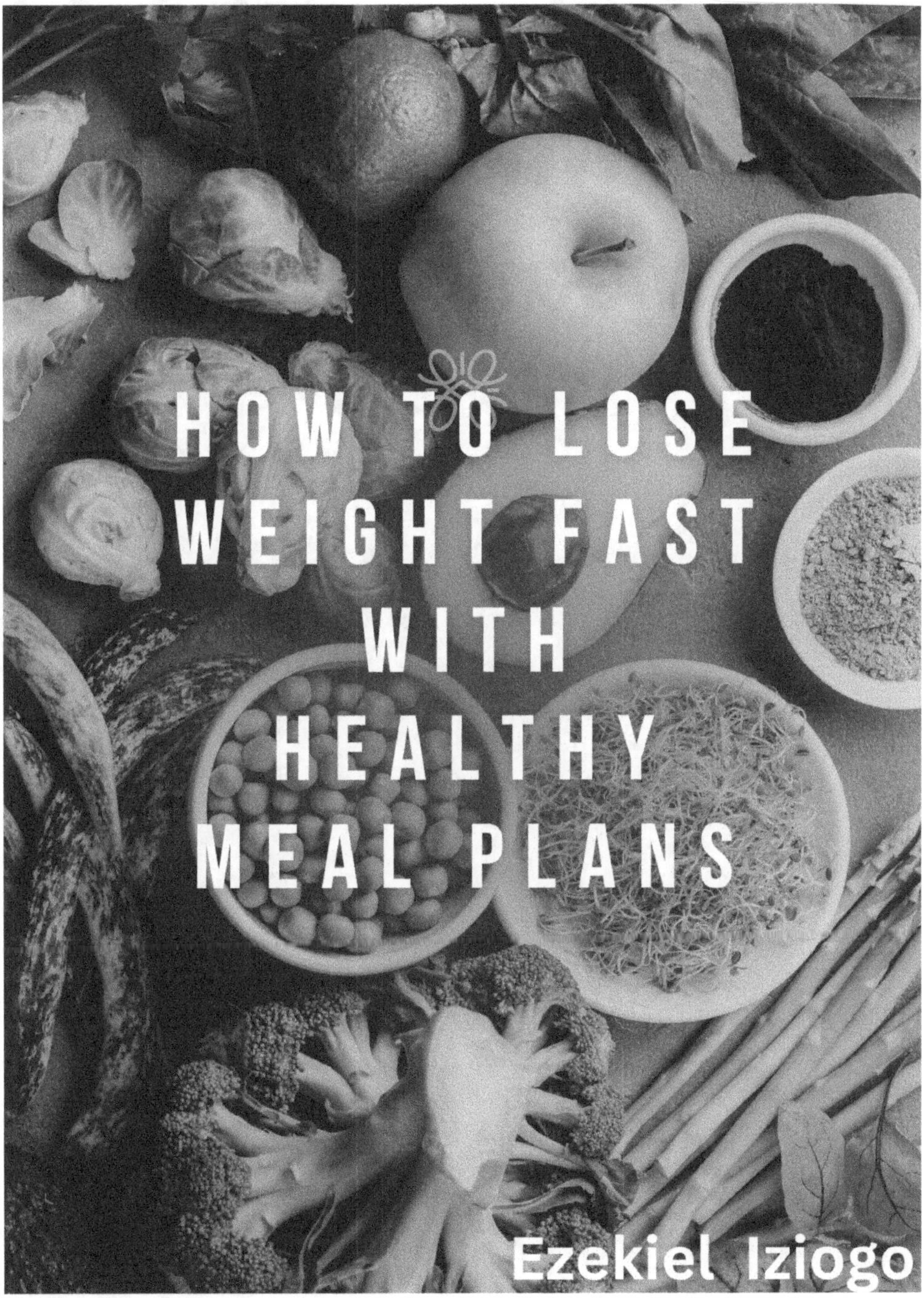

# HOW TO LOSE WEIGHT FAST WITH HEALTHY MEAL PLANS

Ezekiel Iziogo

# How to Lose Weight Fast with Healthy Meal Plans

# TABLE OF CONTENTS

## Introduction

- **Welcome Message**
  - Brief introduction to the ebook's purpose.
  - Highlight the importance of healthy meal planning in weight loss.
- **The Science Behind Weight Loss**
  - Overview of how weight loss works (calories in vs. calories out).
  - The role of metabolism and nutrition in weight management.
- **Why Healthy Meal Plans?**
  - The benefits of structured eating.
  - How meal planning prevents unhealthy eating habits.

## Chapter 1: Understanding Your Weight Loss Goals

- **Setting Realistic Goals**
  - Importance of setting achievable weight loss targets.
  - How to calculate your ideal weight and caloric needs.
- **Tracking Progress**
  - Tips on monitoring your weight loss journey.
  - The value of keeping a food journal or using apps.

## Chapter 2: The Foundations of a Healthy Diet

- **Macronutrients Explained**
  - Overview of proteins, carbohydrates, and fats.
  - The role of each macronutrient in weight loss.

# Chapter 5: Overcoming Common Weight Loss Challenges

- **Dealing with Cravings and Emotional Eating**
  - Techniques to manage and overcome cravings.
  - Strategies for handling emotional eating triggers.
- **Breaking Through Weight Loss Plateaus**
  - Understanding why plateaus happen.
  - Tips for adjusting your meal plan to restart weight loss.
- **Staying Motivated**
  - How to maintain motivation over the long term.
  - The role of support systems and accountability partners.

# Chapter 6: Long-Term Weight Management

- **Transitioning to Maintenance**
  - How to adjust your meal plan once you've reached your goal weight.
  - Tips for maintaining weight loss and avoiding regain.
- **Healthy Habits for Life**
  - Incorporating exercise and active living into your routine.
  - Mindful eating practices for long-term success.

# Chapter 7: Frequently Asked Questions (FAQs)

- **Common Questions About Meal Planning and Weight Loss**
  - Addressing typical concerns and misconceptions.
  - Practical advice based on real-world experiences.

# Conclusion

- **Final Thoughts**

- o   Recap of key points covered in the ebook.
  - o   Encouragement to start implementing the meal plans and tips provided.
- **Call to Action**
  - o   Invite readers to connect with you on social media or through your website for additional support and resources.

## Appendices

- **Appendix A: Grocery Shopping List**
  - o   A comprehensive list of ingredients needed for the meal plans.
- **Appendix B: Meal Plan Templates**
  - o   Blank templates for readers to create their own meal plans.
- **Appendix C: Additional Resources**
  - o   Recommended books, websites, and apps for further reading and tools.

# Introduction

## Welcome Message

Welcome to **"How to Lose Weight Fast with Healthy Meal Plans"** – your comprehensive guide to achieving your weight loss goals through thoughtful, nutritious meal planning. Whether you're just starting your journey or you've been on the path for a while, this ebook is designed to be your roadmap to success.

In today's fast-paced world, many people struggle with weight management, not for lack of trying but often due to the overwhelming amount of conflicting information available. This ebook aims to cut through the noise and provide you with practical, evidence-based strategies that will help you lose weight in a healthy, sustainable way.

Weight loss isn't just about eating less; it's about eating right. It's about nourishing your body with the foods it needs to function optimally while also creating a calorie deficit that allows for weight loss. With the right meal plan, you can achieve your weight loss goals without feeling deprived or overwhelmed. This ebook is here to show you how.

# The Purpose of This Ebook

The purpose of this ebook is to provide you with a clear, actionable plan to lose weight by focusing on healthy eating habits. We'll explore the science behind weight loss, the critical role that nutrition plays, and how you can create and stick to meal plans that are both satisfying and effective.

We'll also address common challenges, such as cravings, emotional eating, and plateaus, providing you with tools and strategies to overcome these obstacles. By the end of this ebook, you'll have a deeper understanding of how your body works, what it needs to thrive, and how you can take control of your weight loss journey.

## The Importance of Healthy Meal Planning in Weight Loss

Healthy meal planning is the cornerstone of successful weight loss. When you plan your meals in advance, you're more likely to make healthier choices, avoid the pitfalls of impulse eating, and ensure that you're getting the right balance of nutrients to support your weight loss goals.

Meal planning helps you stay organized and focused. It eliminates the guesswork, reduces stress, and saves time and money. More importantly, it empowers you to take control of your eating habits, which is essential for long-term weight loss success.

In this ebook, we'll guide you through the process of creating effective meal plans that suit your lifestyle and preferences. You'll learn how to build balanced meals, choose the right ingredients, and prepare your food in a way that supports your weight loss goals. Whether you're cooking for yourself or a family, you'll find practical tips and delicious recipes that make healthy eating enjoyable and sustainable.

## The Science Behind Weight Loss

### Calories In vs. Calories Out

At its core, weight loss is about creating a calorie deficit – that is, consuming fewer calories than your body needs to maintain its current weight. This concept is often summarized as "calories in vs. calories out." When you eat fewer calories than your body burns, your body turns to its fat stores for energy, resulting in weight loss.

However, while the basic principle of calorie balance is simple, the process of achieving it can be more complex. It involves not only reducing calorie intake but also choosing the right types of calories. Not all calories are created equal; the source of your calories – whether from carbohydrates, fats, or proteins – can affect how your body processes them, how full you feel after eating, and how much energy you have throughout the day.

## The Role of Metabolism

Your metabolism plays a critical role in weight loss. Metabolism refers to the chemical processes that occur within your body to maintain life, including the conversion of food into energy. Your basal metabolic rate (BMR) is the number of calories your body needs to perform basic functions like breathing, circulating blood, and maintaining body temperature.

Several factors influence your metabolism, including your age, gender, muscle mass, and activity level. Generally, people with more muscle mass have higher metabolisms because muscle tissue burns more calories at rest than fat tissue. This is why strength training is often recommended as part of a weight loss plan – building muscle can help boost your metabolism and increase the number of calories your body burns, even when you're not exercising.

## Nutrition and Weight Management

Nutrition is the foundation of weight management. The foods you eat not only provide the calories your body needs but also the nutrients it requires to function properly. A well-balanced diet is essential for maintaining energy levels, supporting metabolic processes, and preventing deficiencies that could sabotage your weight loss efforts.

Different nutrients have different effects on your body. For example, protein is particularly important for weight loss because it helps build and repair muscle tissue, keeps you feeling full, and has a higher thermic effect – meaning your body burns more calories digesting protein than it does digesting carbohydrates or fats. On the other hand, too much sugar or refined carbohydrates can lead to spikes and crashes in blood sugar levels, making you feel hungry and tired, which can lead to overeating.

In this ebook, we'll delve deeper into the nutritional aspects of weight loss, exploring how to choose foods that are not only low in calories but also high in essential nutrients. You'll learn how to create balanced meals that support your weight loss goals while keeping you satisfied and energized.

## Why Healthy Meal Plans?

### The Benefits of Structured Eating

Structured eating through meal planning offers numerous benefits for weight loss. When you plan your meals, you're more likely to make thoughtful, healthy choices rather than relying on convenience foods that are often high in calories, fat, and sugar. Meal planning also helps you control portion sizes, reduce food waste, and save money by avoiding last-minute takeout or fast food.

Moreover, meal planning allows you to ensure that your diet is balanced and varied. You can plan meals that include a wide range of foods, ensuring that you get all the nutrients your body needs to stay healthy while losing weight. It also allows you to incorporate foods you enjoy into your diet, making it easier to stick to your weight loss plan in the long term.

## Preventing Unhealthy Eating Habits

One of the biggest challenges people face when trying to lose weight is the temptation to eat unhealthy foods. Whether it's a busy schedule, stress, or simply lack of preparation, it's easy to fall into the habit of grabbing whatever is convenient – often at the expense of your health and weight loss goals.

Meal planning helps you avoid these pitfalls by ensuring that you always have healthy, satisfying meals and snacks on hand. When you know what you're going to eat ahead of time, you're less likely to reach for junk food or overeat. Instead, you can focus on nourishing your body with the foods it needs to thrive.

In this ebook, we'll provide you with practical tips and strategies for meal planning, as well as a variety of delicious, healthy recipes to get you started. Whether you're new to meal planning or looking to refine your approach, you'll find everything you need to create a successful, sustainable meal plan that helps you reach your weight loss goals.

# Conclusion

The introduction chapter sets the stage for the rest of the ebook, giving you a solid foundation in the principles of weight loss and the importance of healthy meal planning. By the time you finish this chapter, you'll be ready to dive into the specifics of creating a meal plan that works for you, with all the tools and knowledge you need to succeed.

In the chapters that follow, we'll take a closer look at how to set your weight loss goals, create balanced meals, and overcome common challenges. We'll also provide you with sample meal plans, recipes, and tips for staying motivated and on track. Whether you're looking to lose a few pounds or make a major transformation, this ebook will be your guide to achieving lasting weight loss through healthy eating.

# Chapter 1: Understanding Your Weight Loss Goals

## Setting Realistic Goals

### Importance of Setting Achievable Weight Loss Targets

When embarking on a weight loss journey, one of the most critical first steps is setting realistic goals. These goals serve as a roadmap, guiding you towards your desired outcomes while keeping you motivated and focused. However, the key to success lies in making sure these goals are both realistic and achievable.

Why is this so important? Because unrealistic goals can lead to frustration, burnout, and ultimately, failure. On the other hand, setting attainable targets provides a sense of accomplishment and progress, which fuels continued effort and commitment.

### Understanding Your Starting Point

Before setting any goals, it's essential to understand where you're starting from. This includes assessing your current weight, body composition, eating habits, and activity level. Many people overlook the importance of this step, but knowing your starting point allows you to set goals that are tailored to your specific needs and circumstances.

## The Dangers of Unrealistic Expectations

Many people set out with the expectation that they can lose a significant amount of weight in a very short period. While rapid weight loss is possible, it's often not sustainable and can lead to a host of problems, including muscle loss, nutritional deficiencies, and metabolic slowdown. Furthermore, when the weight inevitably returns, it can lead to feelings of failure and frustration, which can derail your progress and motivation.

Instead, aim for a gradual, steady weight loss of about 1-2 pounds per week. This rate is generally considered safe and sustainable, allowing your body to adjust to the changes without compromising your health. Remember, the goal is not just to lose weight but to maintain that loss over the long term.

## SMART Goals Framework

A helpful tool for setting realistic and achievable goals is the SMART framework, which stands for Specific, Measurable, Achievable, Relevant, and Time-bound. Let's break down how to apply this framework to your weight loss goals:

- **Specific**: Your goal should be clear and specific. Instead of saying, "I want to lose weight," specify how much weight you want to lose and by when. For example, "I want to lose 10 pounds in the next 8 weeks."

- **Measurable**: You should be able to track your progress. This could be through regular weigh-ins, body measurements, or tracking your food intake and exercise.
- **Achievable**: Your goal should be realistic, given your current lifestyle, resources, and time. Losing 50 pounds in a month is not achievable, but losing 5-10 pounds in that time might be.
- **Relevant**: Your goal should be meaningful and aligned with your broader life goals. Ask yourself why you want to lose weight. Is it for health reasons, to improve your self-esteem, or to prepare for an event? Understanding your motivation will help you stay committed.
- **Time-bound**: Set a deadline for your goal. This creates a sense of urgency and helps you stay focused. For example, "I want to lose 10 pounds by December 1st."

## How to Calculate Your Ideal Weight and Caloric Needs

Once you've set your weight loss goals, the next step is to calculate your ideal weight and caloric needs. Understanding these numbers will help you create a plan that is tailored to your body's requirements, ensuring that you're losing weight in a healthy and sustainable way.

# Calculating Your Ideal Weight

There are various methods to estimate your ideal weight, but it's important to remember that these are just guidelines. Your ideal weight should be based on a combination of factors, including your height, body composition, and overall health.

One commonly used tool is the **Body Mass Index (BMI)**, which is a simple calculation based on your height and weight. The BMI categories are:

- Underweight: BMI below 18.5
- Normal weight: BMI 18.5 - 24.9
- Overweight: BMI 25 - 29.9
- Obese: BMI 30 and above

While BMI can provide a general idea of whether you're within a healthy weight range, it doesn't take into account factors like muscle mass, bone density, and distribution of fat. Therefore, it's not always the best indicator of health for everyone. For a more accurate assessment, you might want to consider your **body fat percentage** or consult with a healthcare professional.

**Tools and Resources for Calculating Ideal Weight:**

- BMI Calculator : Provided by the CDC, this online tool can help you quickly calculate your BMI.
- **Body Fat Percentage Calculators**: Devices like skinfold calipers, bioelectrical impedance scales,

and DEXA scans can provide a more detailed analysis of your body composition.

## Determining Your Daily Caloric Needs

To lose weight, you need to create a calorie deficit, meaning you consume fewer calories than your body burns. But how many calories should you be eating? This can be determined by calculating your **Total Daily Energy Expenditure (TDEE)**, which is the total number of calories your body needs to maintain its current weight, factoring in all activities.

1. **Calculate Your Basal Metabolic Rate (BMR)**: Your BMR is the number of calories your body needs to perform basic functions like breathing and digestion. There are several formulas to calculate BMR, with the **Mifflin-St Jeor Equation** being one of the most commonly used:

   - For men: BMR = 88.36 + (13.4 x weight in kg) + (4.8 x height in cm) - (5.7 x age in years)
   - For women: BMR = 447.6 + (9.2 x weight in kg) + (3.1 x height in cm) - (4.3 x age in years)

2. **Estimate Your Activity Level**: Next, multiply your BMR by an activity factor to estimate your TDEE. The activity factors are:

   - Sedentary (little or no exercise): BMR x 1.2

- Lightly active (light exercise/sports 1-3 days/week): BMR x 1.375
    - Moderately active (moderate exercise/sports 3-5 days/week): BMR x 1.55
    - Very active (hard exercise/sports 6-7 days a week): BMR x 1.725
    - Super active (very hard exercise/physical job): BMR x 1.9
3. **Creating a Calorie Deficit**: Once you know your TDEE, you can create a calorie deficit by reducing your calorie intake, increasing your physical activity, or both. A common recommendation is to aim for a deficit of 500-1,000 calories per day, which should result in a weight loss of about 1-2 pounds per week.

**Tools and Resources for Calculating Caloric Needs:**

- TDEE Calculator : An online tool that can help you estimate your daily caloric needs based on your BMR and activity level.
- MyFitnessPal : A popular app that tracks your daily caloric intake and provides insights into your eating habits.

## Tracking Progress

Monitoring your progress is crucial to achieving your weight loss goals. It not only helps you stay motivated but also allows you to make necessary adjustments to your plan. Whether you're tracking your weight, body measurements, or dietary habits, consistency is key.

**Tips on Monitoring Your Weight Loss Journey**

1. **Regular Weigh-Ins**: Weighing yourself regularly, ideally at the same time each day, can help you track your progress. However, keep in mind that weight can fluctuate due to various factors, including water retention, hormonal changes, and muscle gain. Don't be discouraged by daily fluctuations; instead, focus on the overall trend over time.

2. **Measure Your Body**: In addition to weighing yourself, consider measuring other aspects of your body, such as your waist, hips, arms, and thighs. Sometimes, even when the scale isn't moving, you may notice changes in your measurements as you lose fat and build muscle.

3. **Take Photos**: Progress photos are a great way to visually track your transformation. Take a photo at the start of your journey and update it every few weeks. This can provide a powerful visual reminder of how far you've come.

4. **Track Your Food Intake**: Keeping a detailed record of what you eat is one of the most effective ways to stay on track. This can help you identify patterns, make healthier choices, and stay within

your calorie limits. You can do this with a traditional food journal or use a digital app for more convenience.

5. **Monitor Your Activity Levels**: Whether you're walking, running, lifting weights, or doing yoga, tracking your physical activity can help you stay motivated and see how your efforts are paying off. Many fitness trackers and apps can sync with your phone to provide detailed reports on your activity levels.

## The Value of Keeping a Food Journal or Using Apps

**Benefits of Keeping a Food Journal:**

1. **Increased Awareness:** Writing down everything you eat and drink makes you more aware of your choices. It forces you to think twice before indulging in unhealthy options and helps you identify patterns that might be hindering your progress.

2. **Accountability:** A food journal serves as a record of your daily choices. Knowing that you'll need to write down everything you consume can be a powerful deterrent to mindless snacking or overeating.

3. **Identifying Triggers:** By tracking what you eat and when, you can identify triggers that lead to unhealthy eating. This could be stress, boredom, social situations, or even certain times of the day. Once you recognize these triggers, you can develop strategies to manage them.

4. **Portion Control:** Keeping a food journal can help you become more mindful of portion sizes. Often, people underestimate how much they eat, and writing it down helps you stay within your caloric limits.

5. **Nutritional Insight:** By recording your meals, you can analyze the nutritional quality of your diet. Are you getting enough protein? Are you consuming too much sugar? A food journal can highlight areas where you might need to make adjustments.

6. **Tracking Progress:** Over time, your food journal can serve as a powerful tool to track your progress. You can look back and see how your eating habits have evolved, which can be motivating as you see the positive changes you've made.

## Using Apps for Tracking:

In today's digital age, there are numerous apps designed to make tracking your food intake and physical activity easier than ever. These apps offer a range of features that can enhance your weight loss journey, providing detailed insights and personalized recommendations.

1. **MyFitnessPal:** One of the most popular apps for tracking food intake and exercise, MyFitnessPal allows you to log your meals, monitor your nutrient intake, and set personalized calorie goals. It also has a large database of foods, making it easy to find and log what you've eaten.

2. **Lose It!:** Similar to MyFitnessPal, Lose It! helps you track your meals, set weight loss goals, and monitor your progress. The app also offers a barcode scanner for quick entry of packaged foods and integrates with various fitness devices.

3. **Noom:** Noom takes a psychological approach to weight loss, focusing on behavior change. The app provides personalized coaching, daily lessons, and tracking tools to help you develop healthier habits and stick to your goals.

4. **Cronometer:** Cronometer is a more detailed app that tracks not just calories but also the full spectrum of nutrients in your diet. It's a great tool if you're interested in ensuring you're meeting all your nutritional needs while losing weight.

5. **Fitbit:** If you use a Fitbit device, the accompanying app allows you to track your physical activity, sleep

patterns, and food intake. It provides a comprehensive view of your overall health, which can be incredibly motivating.

6. **Samsung Health/Apple Health:** Both of these apps offer basic tracking features for food, exercise, and sleep. They can be integrated with other health apps and devices to give you a complete picture of your daily habits.

## Overcoming Common Challenges in Goal Setting and Tracking

As with any journey, the road to weight loss is not without its challenges. Recognizing these obstacles and having strategies in place to overcome them is essential for long-term success.

### Challenge 1: Unrealistic Expectations

One of the most common challenges people face when setting weight loss goals is unrealistic expectations. It's easy to get caught up in the desire for quick results, but setting goals that are too ambitious can lead to disappointment and burnout.

**Solution:** Revisit the SMART goals framework and adjust your targets to be more realistic. Remember that sustainable weight loss is a marathon, not a sprint.

Celebrate small victories along the way and keep the bigger picture in mind.

## Challenge 2: Plateaus

Weight loss plateaus can be frustrating and discouraging. After initial success, it's common for progress to slow down or stall completely. This can happen for a variety of reasons, including metabolic adaptation, water retention, or simply needing to adjust your calorie intake or exercise routine.

**Solution:** Don't panic. Plateaus are a normal part of the weight loss process. To overcome them, consider varying your exercise routine, adjusting your calorie intake, or focusing on other aspects of health, such as strength and flexibility. Sometimes, simply giving your body a break can help you push past a plateau.

## Challenge 3: Emotional Eating

Emotional eating is a significant barrier to weight loss for many people. Whether it's stress, sadness, boredom, or celebration, emotions can drive us to eat even when we're not physically hungry.

**Solution:** Develop strategies to manage emotional eating, such as finding alternative coping mechanisms like exercise, meditation, or talking to a friend. Keeping a food journal can also help you identify patterns and triggers, so you can address the root cause of emotional eating.

### Challenge 4: Lack of Time

Busy schedules can make it difficult to stick to a meal plan or find time to exercise. When life gets hectic, it's easy to fall back into unhealthy habits.

**Solution:** Time management is key. Plan your meals ahead of time, prepare food in batches, and schedule your workouts just like you would any other important appointment. Even short, 10-15 minute exercise sessions can be effective if you're consistent.

### Challenge 5: Social Pressure

Social events, gatherings, and peer pressure can make it challenging to stick to your weight loss goals. Whether it's a family dinner, a night out with friends, or holiday celebrations, these situations often involve food and drinks that can derail your progress.

**Solution:** Plan ahead for social situations. Decide in advance what you'll eat, bring a healthy dish to share, or politely decline foods that don't align with your goals. It's also important to communicate your goals with friends and family so they can support you rather than tempt you.

## Maintaining Motivation Throughout Your Journey

Staying motivated is crucial to achieving long-term weight loss success. Motivation can wane over time, especially when progress is slow or challenges arise. Here are some strategies to keep your motivation high:

1. **Set Short-Term Goals:** In addition to your long-term weight loss goal, set smaller, short-term goals that you can achieve along the way. This could be losing the first 5 pounds, completing a fitness challenge, or sticking to your meal plan for a week. Celebrating these smaller milestones can keep you motivated and on track.

2. **Find a Support System:** Having a support system can make all the difference. Whether it's a friend, family member, or online community, sharing your journey with others can provide encouragement, accountability, and motivation.

3. **Visualize Your Success:** Visualization is a powerful tool for staying motivated. Take time each day to imagine yourself achieving your weight loss goals. Picture how you'll feel, how you'll look, and how your life will improve. This positive reinforcement can help keep you focused and driven.

4. **Reward Yourself:** Set up a reward system for reaching your goals. It's important to reward yourself in ways that don't involve food, such as treating yourself to a new outfit, a spa day, or a fun

activity you've been wanting to try.

5. **Stay Positive:** Weight loss can be a challenging journey, and it's normal to experience setbacks along the way. When you encounter obstacles, try to stay positive and remind yourself why you started. Focus on the progress you've made rather than the setbacks.

6. **Reevaluate and Adjust as Needed:** Your goals and plans may need to be adjusted as you progress. If you find that something isn't working, don't be afraid to make changes. Flexibility is key to long-term success.

## Conclusion

Setting and understanding your weight loss goals is a crucial step in your journey toward a healthier, happier you. By taking the time to set realistic, achievable targets, calculate your ideal weight and caloric needs, and track your progress effectively, you're laying the foundation for success.

Remember, weight loss is a journey, not a destination. It's about making sustainable changes that you can maintain for life. As you continue through this ebook, you'll gain the knowledge, tools, and confidence to create healthy meal plans that support your goals and help you achieve lasting results.

# Chapter 2: The Foundations of a Healthy Diet

## Macronutrients Explained

Understanding the basics of nutrition is essential for anyone on a weight loss journey. One of the first concepts to grasp is the role of macronutrients—proteins, carbohydrates, and fats—in your diet. These three components are the primary sources of energy for your body and play unique roles in supporting your health, metabolism, and weight loss efforts.

### Overview of Proteins, Carbohydrates, and Fats

1. **Proteins: The Building Blocks of Life**

   Proteins are essential for growth, repair, and maintenance of body tissues. They are made up of amino acids, which are the building blocks your body uses to create muscle, skin, enzymes, and hormones. In the context of weight loss, protein plays a critical role in maintaining muscle mass while you shed fat. This is important because muscle tissue burns more calories than fat, even at rest.

   - **Sources of Protein:** Lean meats, poultry, fish, eggs, dairy products, legumes, nuts, and seeds are excellent sources of protein.

- **Protein's Role in Weight Loss:** Protein has a high thermic effect, meaning your body burns more calories digesting protein than it does with fats or carbohydrates. It also helps to keep you feeling full and satisfied, reducing the likelihood of overeating.

2. **Key Point:** Aim to include a source of protein in each meal to support muscle maintenance and satiety.

3. **Carbohydrates: Your Body's Preferred Energy Source**

Carbohydrates are your body's primary energy source. They are broken down into glucose, which fuels your brain, muscles, and other vital organs. Carbohydrates are divided into two main types: simple (sugars) and complex (starches and fiber). Complex carbohydrates, which include whole grains, vegetables, and legumes, are digested more slowly, providing a steady release of energy and keeping you full for longer.

- **Sources of Carbohydrates:** Whole grains (like oats, brown rice, quinoa), fruits, vegetables, legumes, and dairy products.
- **Carbohydrates and Weight Loss:** While carbohydrates often get a bad rap in weight loss circles, they are an essential part of a balanced diet. The key is to choose

high-quality, nutrient-dense carbohydrates and to manage portion sizes.

4. **Key Point:** Opt for complex carbohydrates over simple ones, and pair them with protein and fat to slow digestion and avoid blood sugar spikes.

5. **Fats: Essential for Health**

   Fats are essential for hormone production, brain function, and absorbing fat-soluble vitamins (A, D, E, and K). Like carbohydrates, fats come in different forms—saturated, unsaturated, and trans fats. Unsaturated fats, which include monounsaturated and polyunsaturated fats, are considered the healthiest and are found in foods like olive oil, avocados, nuts, and fatty fish.

   - **Sources of Fats:** Avocados, olive oil, nuts, seeds, fatty fish (like salmon and mackerel), and full-fat dairy products.
   - **Fats and Weight Loss:** Healthy fats can be part of a weight loss diet when consumed in moderation. They are calorie-dense, so portion control is key. Including fats in your meals can also increase satiety, helping you feel full and satisfied.

6. **Key Point:** Don't shy away from fats, but focus on healthy sources and be mindful of portions to manage your calorie intake effectively.

# The Role of Each Macronutrient in Weight Loss

Balancing your intake of proteins, carbohydrates, and fats is crucial for weight loss. Each macronutrient plays a unique role in supporting your metabolism, energy levels, and overall health.

- **Protein's Role:** As mentioned earlier, protein supports muscle mass, which is critical for maintaining a healthy metabolism. It also helps to reduce hunger and cravings, making it easier to stick to your calorie goals.

- **Carbohydrate's Role:** Carbohydrates are your body's preferred energy source, especially during physical activity. They fuel your workouts, which are an important part of any weight loss plan. Complex carbohydrates, in particular, provide sustained energy and help to regulate blood sugar levels.

- **Fat's Role:** Fats are essential for hormone production, brain function, and the absorption of certain vitamins. Including healthy fats in your diet can help to keep you satisfied and reduce the likelihood of overeating.

**Balance is Key:** Rather than focusing on eliminating one macronutrient, aim for a balanced approach. A typical macronutrient distribution for weight loss might be around 30-40% protein, 30-40% carbohydrates, and 20-30% fat. However, individual needs can vary, so it's important to find a ratio that works best for your body and lifestyle.

# Micronutrients and Their Importance

While macronutrients are the primary focus of most diets, micronutrients—vitamins and minerals—are equally important. These nutrients are needed in smaller amounts but are essential for overall health and well-being. They support everything from your immune system and bone health to energy production and metabolism.

## Essential Vitamins and Minerals for Weight Loss

1. **Vitamin D:**

   - **Importance:** Vitamin D plays a key role in calcium absorption, bone health, and immune function. It may also influence weight loss by affecting fat storage and hormone regulation.
   - **Sources:** Sunlight, fatty fish, fortified dairy products, and egg yolks.
   - **Note:** Many people are deficient in vitamin D, especially during the winter months. Consider getting your levels checked and taking a supplement if needed.

2. **Calcium:**

- **Importance:** Calcium is essential for strong bones and teeth, but it also plays a role in muscle function, nerve transmission, and blood clotting. Some studies suggest that calcium may help with fat loss, particularly around the midsection.
- **Sources:** Dairy products, leafy green vegetables, fortified plant-based milks, and tofu.

3. **Iron:**

- **Importance:** Iron is crucial for producing hemoglobin, the protein in red blood cells that carries oxygen to your tissues. Without enough iron, you may feel fatigued and weak, which can hinder your weight loss efforts.
- **Sources:** Red meat, poultry, fish, lentils, beans, spinach, and fortified cereals.
- **Note:** Iron absorption is enhanced by vitamin C, so pair iron-rich foods with citrus fruits, tomatoes, or bell peppers for better absorption.

4. **Magnesium:**

- **Importance:** Magnesium is involved in over 300 biochemical reactions in the body, including energy production, muscle function, and blood sugar regulation. Adequate magnesium levels can help prevent muscle cramps and support a healthy metabolism.

- ○ **Sources:** Nuts, seeds, whole grains, leafy green vegetables, and legumes.

5. **B Vitamins:**

   - ○ **Importance:** The B vitamins, including B12, B6, and folate, are essential for energy production, brain function, and DNA synthesis. They also play a role in metabolizing carbohydrates, fats, and proteins.
   - ○ **Sources:** Meat, poultry, fish, eggs, dairy products, whole grains, and leafy greens.
   - ○ **Note:** Vegans and vegetarians may need to supplement with vitamin B12, as it is primarily found in animal products.

6. **Zinc:**

   - ○ **Importance:** Zinc is important for immune function, wound healing, and protein synthesis. It also plays a role in hormone production, including the regulation of appetite-controlling hormones.
   - ○ **Sources:** Meat, shellfish, legumes, seeds, nuts, and whole grains.

## How to Ensure Your Diet Is Balanced and Nutrient-Rich

Achieving a balanced, nutrient-rich diet doesn't have to be complicated. By focusing on whole, unprocessed foods and incorporating a variety of different food groups, you can ensure that you're getting the vitamins and minerals your body needs to function optimally.

1. **Eat a Rainbow:** Aim to include a variety of colorful fruits and vegetables in your diet. Different colors represent different nutrients, so the more variety, the better.

2. **Incorporate Whole Foods:** Focus on whole grains, lean proteins, healthy fats, and plenty of fruits and vegetables. Whole foods are less processed and contain more nutrients than their refined counterparts.

3. **Consider Supplementation:** While it's best to get your nutrients from food, there are times when supplementation may be necessary, such as during pregnancy, if you have a medical condition, or if you follow a restrictive diet. Consult with a healthcare provider to determine if supplements are right for you.

4. **Listen to Your Body:** Pay attention to how your body feels after eating certain foods. If you notice that you feel sluggish, bloated, or unwell after eating certain foods, it may be worth exploring potential food sensitivities or allergies.

# Hydration and Weight Loss

Hydration is often overlooked in weight loss discussions, but it plays a crucial role in your overall health and weight management. Water is involved in nearly every bodily function, from digestion and nutrient absorption to temperature regulation and joint lubrication.

## The Importance of Water Intake

1. **Supports Metabolism:** Drinking water can temporarily boost your metabolism by 24-30%. This effect, known as thermogenesis, can help you burn more calories throughout the day.

2. **Promotes Satiety:** Drinking water before meals can help you feel fuller, reducing your overall calorie intake. In one study, participants who drank water before a meal ate an average of 75 fewer calories during that meal.

3. **Aids Digestion:** Water is essential for the digestive process. It helps break down food so that your body can absorb nutrients effectively and prevents constipation by softening stool and promoting regular bowel movements.

4. **Detoxification:** Water helps flush out toxins and waste products from your body through urine and sweat. Proper hydration supports kidney function

and helps keep your urinary tract healthy.

5. **Improves Exercise Performance:** Staying hydrated enhances your physical performance. Dehydration can lead to decreased endurance, strength, and overall exercise performance, making it harder to achieve your weight loss goals.

## How Dehydration Can Impact Your Weight Loss Efforts

1. **Decreased Metabolism:** Dehydration can slow down your metabolism. When your body is low on fluids, it can't effectively process and utilize nutrients, which can impede your weight loss efforts.

2. **Increased Appetite:** Sometimes, your body can confuse thirst with hunger. This can lead to overeating when a glass of water might have sufficed. Staying hydrated helps you distinguish between true hunger and dehydration.

3. **Reduced Exercise Capacity:** Dehydration can impair your physical performance, making workouts feel more challenging and less effective. If you're unable to exercise at your best, it can affect your overall weight loss progress.

4. **Fatigue and Mood Swings:** Inadequate hydration can lead to fatigue, mood swings, and decreased motivation. Feeling tired or irritable can make it harder to stick to your diet and exercise routine.

## Tips for Staying Hydrated

1. **Drink Water Regularly:** Aim to drink water throughout the day, not just when you're thirsty. A general recommendation is about 8 glasses (2 liters) of water per day, but individual needs may vary based on activity level, climate, and overall health.

2. **Incorporate Hydrating Foods:** Many fruits and vegetables have high water content and can contribute to your daily hydration needs. Examples include cucumbers, watermelon, oranges, and strawberries.

3. **Carry a Reusable Water Bottle:** Having a water bottle with you at all times can serve as a constant reminder to drink more water. Choose a bottle that is easy to carry and refill.

4. **Set Hydration Goals:** Use apps or reminders to track your water intake and set daily hydration goals. This can help you stay accountable and ensure you're meeting your needs.

5. **Flavor Your Water:** If you find plain water boring, add natural flavorings like lemon slices, cucumber, or mint leaves. This can make drinking water more enjoyable and encourage you to drink more.

6. **Monitor Your Hydration Status:** Pay attention to signs of dehydration, such as dark yellow urine, dry skin, or dizziness. Adjust your water intake accordingly if you notice these symptoms.

# Conclusion

Understanding the foundations of a healthy diet is crucial for successful weight loss. By grasping the roles of macronutrients and micronutrients and recognizing the importance of hydration, you can create a balanced, nutrient-rich diet that supports your weight loss goals and overall health.

Balancing proteins, carbohydrates, and fats while ensuring you get essential vitamins and minerals will help your body function optimally and sustain energy levels. Staying hydrated is equally important, as it affects metabolism, appetite, and exercise performance.

As you progress through your weight loss journey, remember that a well-rounded diet, combined with regular physical activity, is key to achieving and maintaining your goals. In the next chapter, we'll dive deeper into creating effective meal plans to support your weight loss efforts and ensure you stay on track.

# Chapter 3: Creating Your Weight Loss Meal Plan

## Building a Balanced Plate

Creating a balanced meal is key to supporting weight loss and maintaining overall health. Understanding how to portion your plate and select the right food groups ensures that you're fueling your body with the nutrients it needs while managing calorie intake.

### Guidelines for Portion Sizes and Food Groups

1. **Portion Sizes:**

   - **Proteins:** Aim for about 3-4 ounces of lean protein per meal. This is roughly the size of a deck of cards. Protein should be the star of your meal, providing the majority of your calorie intake.
   - **Carbohydrates:** Include a portion of complex carbohydrates, such as whole grains or starchy vegetables, about the size of your fist. This helps provide sustained energy without excess calories.
   - **Fats:** Incorporate a small amount of healthy fats, such as a tablespoon of olive oil, a handful of nuts, or a quarter of an avocado. Fats are calorie-dense, so moderation is key.

- **Vegetables:** Fill half of your plate with non-starchy vegetables. These are low in calories and high in fiber, helping you feel full and satisfied.

2. **Food Groups:**

   - **Lean Proteins:** Chicken breast, turkey, fish, tofu, legumes, and low-fat dairy products.
   - **Complex Carbohydrates:** Quinoa, brown rice, whole-wheat pasta, sweet potatoes, and oats.
   - **Healthy Fats:** Olive oil, avocado, nuts, seeds, and fatty fish.
   - **Vegetables:** Spinach, kale, broccoli, bell peppers, carrots, and cauliflower.
   - **Fruits:** Berries, apples, oranges, and bananas can be included in moderation for natural sweetness and nutrients.

**Example Plate:** For a balanced dinner, you might have a grilled chicken breast (protein), a serving of quinoa (carbohydrate), a side of steamed broccoli (vegetable), and a small drizzle of olive oil (fat).

## How to Create Meals that Satisfy Hunger and Support Weight Loss

1. **Prioritize Protein and Fiber:** Meals high in protein and fiber help you stay full longer. Incorporate sources of lean protein and high-fiber vegetables and grains into your meals. This combination helps

regulate appetite and reduces the likelihood of overeating.

2. **Incorporate Healthy Fats:** While fats are calorie-dense, they also play a crucial role in satiety. Including a small amount of healthy fats can help keep you feeling full and satisfied. Examples include adding avocado to your salad or a sprinkle of nuts on your yogurt.

3. **Use Spices and Herbs:** Flavoring your meals with spices and herbs can enhance taste without adding extra calories or sodium. Try using garlic, cumin, turmeric, basil, and rosemary to boost flavor and nutritional value.

4. **Stay Hydrated:** Drinking water with your meals aids digestion and can help prevent overeating. Sometimes, thirst is mistaken for hunger, so staying hydrated is crucial for managing appetite.

5. **Plan Balanced Snacks:** If you need a snack between meals, opt for options that include protein and fiber. Examples include a handful of almonds, Greek yogurt with fruit, or carrot sticks with hummus.

# Meal Planning for Success

Effective meal planning can simplify your weight loss journey and ensure you stay on track with your goals. By preparing meals ahead of time and customizing your plan to fit your needs, you can make healthy eating more manageable.

## Tips for Planning Meals Ahead of Time

1. **Create a Weekly Meal Schedule:** Outline your meals for the week, including breakfast, lunch, dinner, and snacks. This helps you stay organized and ensures that you have a plan for every meal.

2. **Prepare a Shopping List:** Based on your meal plan, create a detailed shopping list. This helps you avoid impulse buys and ensures that you have all the ingredients you need.

3. **Batch Cook and Prep:** Spend a few hours each week preparing and cooking meals in bulk. This can include roasting vegetables, cooking grains, and grilling proteins. Store these items in the refrigerator or freezer for easy access throughout the week.

4. **Use Storage Containers:** Invest in quality storage containers to keep your prepped meals fresh. Portion out your meals into individual containers for

easy grab-and-go options.

5. **Mix and Match:** To keep meals interesting and prevent boredom, mix and match different proteins, carbohydrates, and vegetables throughout the week. This adds variety and ensures that you're getting a wide range of nutrients.

## How to Customize Meal Plans Based on Personal Preferences and Dietary Needs

1. **Consider Dietary Restrictions:** If you have food allergies, intolerances, or specific dietary needs (e.g., gluten-free, vegan), adjust your meal plan accordingly. Substitute ingredients that fit your dietary requirements while maintaining nutritional balance.

2. **Account for Taste Preferences:** Tailor your meal plan to include foods you enjoy. If you dislike certain vegetables or grains, swap them out for alternatives that you prefer. Enjoying your meals increases the likelihood of sticking to your plan.

3. **Adjust Portion Sizes:** Depending on your activity level, metabolism, and weight loss goals, you may need to adjust portion sizes. For example, someone with a higher activity level may require larger portions of carbohydrates compared to

someone who is less active.

4. **Include Occasional Treats:** Allowing yourself occasional treats can help prevent feelings of deprivation. Plan for these treats in advance and ensure they fit within your overall calorie and nutritional goals.

5. **Seek Professional Guidance:** If you're unsure how to create a meal plan that meets your specific needs, consider consulting with a registered dietitian or nutritionist. They can provide personalized advice and help you develop a plan that supports your weight loss goals.

## Sample 7-Day Weight Loss Meal Plan

To help you get started, here's a sample 7-day meal plan that includes breakfast, lunch, dinner, and snacks. Feel free to adjust the meals based on your preferences and dietary needs.

### Day 1:

- **Breakfast:** Greek yogurt with fresh berries and a sprinkle of chia seeds.
- **Lunch:** Grilled chicken salad with mixed greens, cherry tomatoes, cucumber, and a light vinaigrette.
- **Dinner:** Baked salmon with quinoa and steamed asparagus.

- **Snack:** Apple slices with almond butter.

## Day 2:

- **Breakfast:** Overnight oats with almond milk, sliced banana, and a dash of cinnamon.
- **Lunch:** Turkey and avocado wrap with whole wheat tortilla and a side of baby carrots.
- **Dinner:** Stir-fried tofu with broccoli, bell peppers, and brown rice.
- **Snack:** A handful of mixed nuts.

## Day 3:

- **Breakfast:** Smoothie with spinach, frozen berries, protein powder, and unsweetened almond milk.
- **Lunch:** Lentil soup with a side salad of mixed greens and a light lemon dressing.
- **Dinner:** Grilled shrimp with sweet potato wedges and a side of sautéed kale.
- **Snack:** Greek yogurt with a drizzle of honey.

## Day 4:

- **Breakfast:** Scrambled eggs with spinach and a slice of whole-grain toast.
- **Lunch:** Quinoa salad with black beans, corn, avocado, and a lime dressing.
- **Dinner:** Chicken stir-fry with mixed vegetables and a side of brown rice.
- **Snack:** Celery sticks with hummus.

# Day 5:

- **Breakfast:** Chia pudding made with almond milk, topped with fresh strawberries.
- **Lunch:** Baked falafel with a side of tabbouleh and a small serving of tzatziki.
- **Dinner:** Turkey meatballs with spaghetti squash and marinara sauce.
- **Snack:** Cottage cheese with pineapple chunks.

# Day 6:

- **Breakfast:** Smoothie bowl with blended spinach, banana, and protein powder, topped with granola and sliced almonds.
- **Lunch:** Grilled vegetable and quinoa bowl with a balsamic glaze.
- **Dinner:** Baked chicken breast with roasted Brussels sprouts and a side of wild rice.
- **Snack:** A pear with a handful of walnuts.

# Day 7:

- **Breakfast:** Avocado toast with a poached egg and a side of mixed fruit.
- **Lunch:** Chickpea salad with cucumber, red onion, bell peppers, and a lemon-tahini dressing.
- **Dinner:** Fish tacos with cabbage slaw and a side of black beans.
- **Snack:** A small handful of dark chocolate chips.

**Recipes and Grocery Lists for Easy Preparation**

To make meal prep easier, here are some basic recipes and grocery lists based on the sample meal plan:

**Recipes:**

1. **Grilled Chicken Salad:**

   ○ **Ingredients:** Chicken breast, mixed greens, cherry tomatoes, cucumber, olive oil, balsamic vinegar.
   ○ **Instructions:** Grill the chicken breast until cooked through. Slice and place on a bed of mixed greens with cherry tomatoes and cucumber. Drizzle with olive oil and balsamic vinegar.

2. **Overnight Oats:**

   ○ **Ingredients:** Rolled oats, almond milk, banana, chia seeds, cinnamon.
   ○ **Instructions:** Combine oats, almond milk, chia seeds, and a sprinkle of cinnamon in a jar. Refrigerate overnight. Top with sliced banana in the morning.

3. **Baked Salmon:**

   ○ **Ingredients:** Salmon filets, lemon, olive oil, salt, pepper.
   ○ **Instructions:** Preheat oven to 375°F (190°C). Place salmon filets on a baking sheet, drizzle with olive oil, and season with salt, pepper, and lemon slices. Bake for

15-20 minutes, or until the salmon flakes easily with a fork. Serve with quinoa and steamed asparagus.

3. **Lentil Soup:**

   - **Ingredients:** Green lentils, onion, carrots, celery, garlic, vegetable broth, diced tomatoes, cumin, salt, pepper.
   - **Instructions:** Sauté onions, carrots, celery, and garlic in a large pot until softened. Add lentils, vegetable broth, diced tomatoes, cumin, salt, and pepper. Simmer for 30-40 minutes until the lentils are tender.

4. **Chicken Stir-Fry:**

   - **Ingredients:** Chicken breast, broccoli, bell peppers, soy sauce, garlic, ginger, olive oil, brown rice.
   - **Instructions:** Cut chicken into strips and cook in a pan with olive oil until browned. Add chopped broccoli and bell peppers, and stir-fry with garlic and ginger. Pour in soy sauce and cook until vegetables are tender. Serve over brown rice.

5. **Chia Pudding:**

   - **Ingredients:** Chia seeds, almond milk, honey, fresh strawberries.
   - **Instructions:** Combine chia seeds and almond milk in a bowl. Stir well and

refrigerate for at least 4 hours or overnight. Top with honey and fresh strawberries before serving.

6. **Fish Tacos:**

   - **Ingredients:** White fish fillets (e.g., cod or tilapia), taco seasoning, corn tortillas, cabbage, lime, cilantro.
   - **Instructions:** Season fish fillets with taco seasoning and bake or grill until cooked through. Shred cabbage and toss with lime juice and chopped cilantro. Serve fish in corn tortillas topped with cabbage slaw.

## Grocery Lists:

## Proteins:

- Chicken breasts
- Salmon filets
- Tofu
- Greek yogurt
- Turkey meatballs
- White fish filets
- Eggs
- Cottage cheese

## Carbohydrates:

- Quinoa
- Brown rice
- Sweet potatoes

- Whole-grain tortillas
- Rolled oats
- Spaghetti squash
- Whole-grain bread

## Fats:

- Olive oil
- Avocado
- Almond butter
- Nuts (almonds, walnuts)
- Chia seeds
- Nut butter

## Vegetables:

- Mixed greens
- Cherry tomatoes
- Cucumber
- Broccoli
- Bell peppers
- Asparagus
- Brussels sprouts
- Kale
- Carrots
- Celery
- Cabbage

## Fruits:

- Berries (strawberries, blueberries)
- Apples

- Bananas
- Pears
- Pineapple chunks
- Lemons
- Oranges

**Other:**

- Almond milk
- Vegetable broth
- Diced tomatoes
- Soy sauce
- Hummus
- Dark chocolate chips
- Honey
- Taco seasoning

# Conclusion

Creating an effective weight loss meal plan involves understanding how to build balanced meals, plan ahead, and customize your approach based on personal preferences and dietary needs. By incorporating a variety of proteins, carbohydrates, fats, and vegetables, and staying hydrated, you can support your weight loss goals while enjoying satisfying and nutritious meals.

The sample 7-day meal plan provided offers a starting point for structuring your meals. Feel free to adjust the recipes and grocery lists based on your taste preferences and dietary requirements. With thoughtful planning and preparation, you can make healthy eating a seamless part of your weight loss journey.

In the next chapter, we'll explore strategies for maintaining your meal plan, overcoming common challenges, and adapting your plan as you progress toward your weight loss goals.

# Chapter 4: Adapting Meal Plans to Your Lifestyle

In today's fast-paced world, adapting meal plans to fit your lifestyle is essential for maintaining a successful weight loss journey. Whether you have a busy schedule, need quick meal ideas, or are navigating social events and dining out, these strategies will help you stay on track without feeling overwhelmed.

## Meal Prep for Busy Schedules

Effective meal prep can save time, reduce stress, and ensure that you always have healthy options readily available. Here's how you can make meal prep work for your busy lifestyle.

### How to Save Time with Batch Cooking and Meal Prep Tips

1. **Plan Your Meals:**

   - **Weekly Planning:** Dedicate some time each week to plan your meals. Outline your breakfast, lunch, dinner, and snacks for the week. Use a meal planning app or a simple spreadsheet to keep track.
   - **Recipe Selection:** Choose recipes that use similar ingredients to simplify shopping and cooking. For example, if you're using chicken

in multiple recipes, buy it in bulk and use it throughout the week.

2. **Grocery Shopping:**

   - **Create a Shopping List:** Based on your meal plan, create a comprehensive shopping list. This helps ensure you have all the ingredients you need and prevents last-minute grocery runs.
   - **Stick to the List:** Avoid impulse buys by sticking to your list. This helps manage your budget and prevents the purchase of unhealthy options.

3. **Batch Cooking:**

   - **Cook in Bulk:** Prepare large quantities of staple items like grains, proteins, and vegetables. For example, cook a big batch of quinoa or brown rice and portion it out for multiple meals.
   - **Use a Slow Cooker or Instant Pot:** These appliances are excellent for preparing large quantities of food with minimal effort. Throw ingredients into the pot, set it, and let it cook while you focus on other tasks.

4. **Portion Control:**

   - **Use Containers:** Invest in high-quality, stackable containers for meal storage.

Portion out meals into individual containers
for easy grab-and-go options.

- o **Label and Date:** Label containers with the
  contents and the date they were prepared.
  This helps keep track of freshness and
  ensures you're eating meals within a safe
  time frame.

5. **Freeze for Convenience:**

- o **Freezer Meals:** Prepare and freeze
  individual portions of meals for easy
  reheating. Soups, stews, and casseroles
  freeze well and can be quickly defrosted and
  reheated.
- o **Label Freezer Bags:** Use freezer bags for
  items like pre-chopped vegetables or
  marinated proteins. Label them with the date
  and contents for easy identification.

**Quick and Easy Recipes for Those on the Go**

1. **Microwavable Veggie and Chicken Wrap:**

- o **Ingredients:** Whole wheat tortilla,
  pre-cooked chicken breast, mixed vegetables
  (e.g., bell peppers, spinach), hummus.
- o **Instructions:** Spread hummus on the tortilla,
  add pre-cooked chicken and vegetables. Roll
  up and microwave for 1-2 minutes, or until
  heated through.

2. **One-Pan Baked Salmon and Vegetables:**

   - **Ingredients:** Salmon filets, cherry tomatoes, zucchini, olive oil, garlic powder.
   - **Instructions:** Place salmon and chopped vegetables on a baking sheet. Drizzle with olive oil and sprinkle with garlic powder. Bake at 375°F (190°C) for 20 minutes or until salmon is cooked through.

3. **Greek Yogurt Parfait:**

   - **Ingredients:** Greek yogurt, granola, fresh berries, honey.
   - **Instructions:** Layer Greek yogurt, granola, and berries in a jar. Drizzle with honey and enjoy it as a quick breakfast or snack.

4. **Quinoa Salad with Chickpeas:**

   - **Ingredients:** Cooked quinoa, canned chickpeas, cherry tomatoes, cucumber, feta cheese, lemon juice.
   - **Instructions:** Combine quinoa, chickpeas, chopped tomatoes, cucumber, and feta cheese in a bowl. Toss with lemon juice and serve.

5. **Smoothie Bowl:**

   - **Ingredients:** Frozen berries, banana, spinach, almond milk, granola.

- Instructions: Blend frozen berries, banana, spinach, and almond milk until smooth. Pour into a bowl and top with granola.

## Eating Out and Staying on Track

Navigating restaurants and social events while staying committed to your weight loss goals can be challenging. Here are strategies to help you make healthier choices and handle special occasions.

## Strategies for Making Healthy Choices at Restaurants

1. **Review Menus in Advance:**

   - **Online Research:** Many restaurants post their menus online. Review the menu ahead of time to identify healthy options and make a decision before you arrive.
   - **Nutritional Information:** Some restaurants provide nutritional information for their dishes. Look for options lower in calories, fats, and sodium.

2. **Choose Wisely:**

   - **Opt for Grilled or Baked Items:** Choose dishes that are grilled, baked, or steamed rather than fried. These cooking methods generally use less oil and are lower in calories.

- Ask for Dressings on the Side: Request dressings and sauces on the side to control the amount you use. This helps you manage calorie intake and avoid extra sugars and fats.

3. **Control Portions:**

- **Share or Save:** Portion sizes at restaurants can be large. Consider sharing a dish with a dining companion or saving half for later. You can also ask for a to-go box at the start of your meal to separate a portion for later.

4. **Focus on Vegetables:**

- **Vegetable Sides:** Choose vegetable-based sides or salads to increase your intake of fiber and nutrients. Ask for steamed or grilled vegetables rather than creamy or fried options.

5. **Stay Hydrated:**

- **Water First:** Drink water before and during your meal. It can help with digestion and reduce the likelihood of overeating.

## How to Handle Social Situations and Special Occasions

1. **Plan Ahead:**

- ○ **Bring a Dish:** If you're attending a potluck or gathering, bring a healthy dish that you can enjoy. This ensures you have a nutritious option available.
- ○ **Communicate Your Needs:** If you're going to a restaurant or event, communicate your dietary preferences or restrictions in advance if possible.

2. **Practice Moderation:**

- ○ **Enjoy in Moderation:** It's okay to indulge occasionally, but do so in moderation. Savor small portions of higher-calorie foods and balance them with healthier choices throughout the day.

3. **Stay Active:**

- ○ **Incorporate Exercise:** Plan to include physical activity on days when you have social events. A brisk walk before or after the event can help offset any extra calories consumed.

4. **Mindful Eating:**

- ○ **Slow Down:** Eat slowly and mindfully. Pay attention to hunger and fullness cues to prevent overeating. Enjoy the company and focus on the social aspects rather than just the food.

5. **Handle Peer Pressure:**

  ○ **Be Assertive:** It's okay to politely decline foods or portions that don't align with your goals. Be confident in your choices and focus on making healthier decisions without feeling pressured.

# Conclusion

Adapting meal plans to fit your lifestyle involves practical strategies for meal prep, quick recipes, and making healthy choices in various situations. By planning ahead, incorporating efficient meal prep techniques, and navigating dining out and social events wisely, you can maintain your weight loss goals while enjoying a balanced and fulfilling life.

The next chapter will explore advanced meal planning strategies and techniques for optimizing your diet and achieving long-term success. Stay tuned for more insights and practical tips to help you continue your weight loss journey.

# Chapter 5: Overcoming Common Weight Loss Challenges

Embarking on a weight loss journey often involves overcoming various challenges. Understanding and addressing these common obstacles can help you stay on track and achieve your goals. This chapter provides strategies for managing cravings and emotional eating, breaking through weight loss plateaus, and maintaining motivation.

## Dealing with Cravings and Emotional Eating

Cravings and emotional eating are significant hurdles for many people trying to lose weight. They can undermine your progress and make it challenging to stick to your meal plan. Here's how to manage and overcome these challenges.

## Techniques to Manage and Overcome Cravings

1. **Identify Triggers:**

   - **Recognize Patterns:** Keep a journal to track when and why you experience cravings. Identifying triggers—such as stress, boredom, or specific times of day—can help you develop strategies to address them.

- **Emotional vs. Physical Hunger:** Learn to distinguish between emotional and physical hunger. Emotional hunger often arises suddenly and is linked to feelings, while physical hunger builds gradually and is satisfied by eating.

2. **Healthy Alternatives:**

   - **Substitute Smartly:** Find healthier alternatives to your cravings. For example, if you crave sweets, opt for fruit or yogurt with a touch of honey instead of sugary snacks.
   - **Mindful Eating:** Practice mindful eating by savoring each bite and focusing on the flavors and textures of your food. This can help you feel more satisfied and reduce the urge to snack mindlessly.

3. **Stay Hydrated:**

   - **Drink Water:** Sometimes cravings are mistaken for thirst. Drink a glass of water when you feel a craving coming on to see if it subsides. Staying hydrated supports overall health and can help manage hunger.

4. **Use Distraction Techniques:**

   - **Engage in Activities:** Distract yourself with activities that keep your mind off cravings, such as going for a walk, reading, or engaging in a hobby.

- **Social Interaction:** Talk to a friend or family member when you're feeling tempted. Social support can provide encouragement and help you stay focused on your goals.

5. **Practice Portion Control:**

- **Controlled Indulgence:** If you choose to indulge in a craving, do so in moderation. Allow yourself a small portion and savor it slowly to avoid overconsumption.

## Strategies for Handling Emotional Eating Triggers

1. **Develop Coping Mechanisms:**

- **Stress Management:** Incorporate stress-reducing techniques such as meditation, deep breathing exercises, or yoga into your routine. Managing stress can reduce emotional eating triggers.
- **Seek Professional Help:** If emotional eating is a significant challenge, consider speaking with a therapist or counselor who specializes in eating disorders or emotional well-being.

2. **Create a Supportive Environment:**

- **Remove Temptations:** Keep unhealthy snacks out of your home. Stock your pantry with nutritious options that support your weight loss goals.

- Build a Support Network: Share your weight loss goals with friends and family. Their support can provide encouragement and accountability.

3. **Establish Healthy Routines:**

   - **Regular Meals:** Eat regular, balanced meals to maintain stable blood sugar levels and reduce the likelihood of emotional eating. Avoid skipping meals, which can lead to overeating later.
   - **Emotional Awareness:** Pay attention to your emotions and address them through healthy coping strategies rather than turning to food for comfort.

# Breaking Through Weight Loss Plateaus

Experiencing a weight loss plateau can be frustrating and discouraging. Understanding why plateaus happen and how to adjust your meal plan can help you overcome these periods of stagnation.

### Understanding Why Plateaus Happen

1. **Metabolic Adaptation:**

   - **Body Adjustment:** As you lose weight, your body's metabolism may slow down to adapt to the new weight. This can reduce the rate of weight loss and result in a plateau.

- ○ **Caloric Needs:** Your caloric needs decrease as you lose weight. A plateau may occur if your calorie intake is no longer aligned with your new weight and activity level.

2. **Changes in Muscle Mass:**

   - ○ **Muscle Growth:** Increased physical activity and strength training can lead to muscle growth. Muscle tissue is denser than fat, which can sometimes mask fat loss on the scale.

3. **Water Retention:**

   - ○ **Temporary Weight Fluctuations:** Factors such as hormonal changes, high sodium intake, or intense exercise can cause temporary water retention, which may affect your weight on the scale.

## Tips for Adjusting Your Meal Plan to Restart Weight Loss

1. **Reassess Caloric Intake:**

   - ○ **Update Caloric Needs:** Recalculate your daily caloric needs based on your current weight and activity level. Adjust your intake accordingly to continue progressing toward your goals.

- **Reduce Portion Sizes:** Consider slightly reducing portion sizes or making healthier food swaps to create a calorie deficit.

2. **Vary Your Exercise Routine:**

   - **Change Workouts:** Introduce variety into your exercise routine to challenge your body in new ways. Incorporate different types of workouts, such as interval training, strength training, or group classes.
   - **Increase Intensity:** Increase the intensity or duration of your workouts to boost calorie burn and break through a plateau.

3. **Monitor Macronutrient Ratios:**

   - **Adjust Macronutrients:** Review your macronutrient distribution (proteins, carbohydrates, and fats) and make adjustments if needed. A shift in macronutrient ratios can help overcome plateaus.

4. **Track Progress Beyond the Scale:**

   - **Measure Other Indicators:** Use other methods to track progress, such as body measurements, clothing fit, or fitness improvements. These indicators can provide motivation and insight when the scale isn't moving.

# Staying Motivated

Maintaining motivation over the long term is crucial for achieving and sustaining weight loss success. Here are strategies to help you stay focused and committed to your goals.

## How to Maintain Motivation Over the Long Term

1. **Set Short-Term Goals:**

   - **Achievable Milestones:** Break your weight loss journey into smaller, manageable goals. Celebrate each milestone to maintain motivation and build momentum.
   - **Track Achievements:** Keep a journal or use an app to track your progress and celebrate your successes, no matter how small.

2. **Stay Accountable:**

   - **Share Your Goals:** Share your goals with friends, family, or a support group. Accountability partners can provide encouragement and help you stay committed.
   - **Regular Check-Ins:** Schedule regular check-ins with yourself or a mentor to assess your progress and make any necessary adjustments to your plan.

3. **Visualize Success:**

- **Create a Vision Board:** Develop a vision board with images and statements that represent your weight loss goals and aspirations. Place it where you can see it daily to stay inspired.
- **Positive Affirmations:** Use positive affirmations to reinforce your commitment and self-belief. Remind yourself of your achievements and the benefits of reaching your goals.

## The Role of Support Systems and Accountability Partners

1. **Build a Support Network:**

   - **Family and Friends:** Surround yourself with supportive individuals who encourage and motivate you. Their support can make a significant difference in your weight loss journey.
   - **Online Communities:** Join online forums or social media groups focused on weight loss and healthy living. Connecting with others who share similar goals can provide inspiration and advice.

2. **Work with a Coach or Dietitian:**

   - **Professional Guidance:** Consider working with a registered dietitian or weight loss

coach who can provide personalized
guidance, support, and accountability.
  - **Regular Sessions:** Schedule regular
    sessions to review your progress, discuss
    challenges, and adjust your plan as needed.
3. **Participate in Group Activities:**

  - **Group Fitness Classes:** Join group fitness
    classes or sports teams to stay motivated
    and engaged. The social aspect of group
    activities can enhance motivation and
    accountability.
  - **Weight Loss Challenges:** Participate in
    weight loss challenges or programs that offer
    structured plans and group support.

# Conclusion

Overcoming weight loss challenges requires a proactive
approach and the ability to adapt to various obstacles. By
managing cravings and emotional eating, addressing
weight loss plateaus, and maintaining motivation, you
can stay on track and achieve your weight loss goals.
Implementing these strategies will help you navigate your
journey with confidence and resilience.

In the next chapter, we will delve into maintaining
long-term weight loss success and creating sustainable
habits for a healthier lifestyle.

# Chapter 6: Long-Term Weight Management

Achieving your weight loss goals is a significant accomplishment, but maintaining your new weight is equally important. This chapter provides strategies for transitioning to weight maintenance, tips for avoiding weight regain, and guidelines for incorporating healthy habits into your daily life.

## Transitioning to Maintenance

Successfully transitioning to a weight maintenance phase involves adjusting your approach to ensure that you sustain your results without reverting to old habits. Here's how to make this transition effectively.

### How to Adjust Your Meal Plan Once You've Reached Your Goal Weight

1. **Recalculate Your Caloric Needs:**

   - **New Caloric Intake:** Once you reach your goal weight, your caloric needs will change. Use a calorie calculator to determine your new daily caloric requirements based on your current weight, age, activity level, and metabolism. Calorie Calculator
   - **Adjust Portion Sizes:** Increase your portion sizes slightly to align with your new caloric

needs. This helps prevent weight regain while still maintaining a balanced diet.

2. **Incorporate More Variety:**

   - **Diversify Your Diet:** Introduce a wider variety of foods into your diet to ensure that you're getting all essential nutrients. Experiment with new recipes and incorporate different fruits, vegetables, proteins, and whole grains.
   - **Moderation:** Enjoy previously restricted foods in moderation. This helps prevent feelings of deprivation and supports long-term adherence to your maintenance plan.

3. **Monitor and Adjust:**

   - **Regular Check-Ins:** Continue to monitor your weight and adjust your meal plan as needed. Regularly weigh yourself or use other methods, such as body measurements or clothing fit, to track your progress.
   - **Flexible Approach:** Be flexible with your meal plan and make adjustments based on your lifestyle and any changes in your activity level or metabolism.

4. **Focus on Balanced Nutrition:**

   - **Nutrient-Rich Foods:** Prioritize nutrient-dense foods that provide vitamins, minerals, and other essential nutrients. Include a variety of vegetables, fruits, lean proteins, whole grains, and healthy fats in your diet.

- o **Avoid Extreme Diets:** Steer clear of extreme diets or restrictive eating patterns that could lead to unhealthy weight fluctuations. Aim for a balanced and sustainable approach to nutrition.

## Tips for Maintaining Weight Loss and Avoiding Regain

1. **Establish a Routine:**

   - o **Consistent Habits:** Develop consistent eating and exercise habits. Maintain a regular meal schedule and incorporate physical activity into your daily routine.
   - o **Healthy Environment:** Create a supportive environment by keeping healthy foods accessible and removing or limiting temptation.

2. **Stay Active:**

   - o **Regular Exercise:** Engage in regular physical activity to support weight maintenance and overall health. Aim for at least 150 minutes of moderate-intensity exercise per week, such as brisk walking or cycling.

- **Strength Training:** Include strength training exercises to build and maintain muscle mass, which can help boost metabolism and support long-term weight management.

3. **Practice Mindful Eating:**

   - **Listen to Your Body:** Pay attention to hunger and fullness cues. Eat slowly and mindfully to enjoy your food and prevent overeating.
   - **Avoid Emotional Eating:** Address emotional triggers without turning to food. Practice stress management techniques and seek support if needed.

4. **Set New Goals:**

   - **Maintain Motivation:** Set new, non-weight-related goals to keep yourself motivated. Focus on improving fitness, trying new activities, or enhancing overall well-being.
   - **Celebrate Success:** Celebrate your achievements and milestones. Recognize and reward yourself for maintaining your weight loss and adopting a healthy lifestyle.

## Healthy Habits for Life

Incorporating healthy habits into your daily routine is key to long-term weight management and overall well-being.

This section explores strategies for maintaining an active lifestyle and practicing mindful eating.

**Incorporating Exercise and Active Living Into Your Routine**

1. **Find Activities You Enjoy:**

   - **Personal Preferences:** Choose physical activities that you enjoy and that fit your lifestyle. Whether it's dancing, hiking, swimming, or playing a sport, finding activities you love can make exercise feel less like a chore.
   - **Variety:** Incorporate a mix of cardiovascular, strength, and flexibility exercises into your routine. Variety helps prevent boredom and keeps your workouts engaging.

2. **Set Realistic Goals:**

   - **Achievable Targets:** Set realistic and attainable exercise goals. Start with small, manageable goals and gradually increase intensity and duration as you progress.
   - **Track Progress:** Use fitness apps or journals to track your exercise routine and progress. Monitoring your activity levels can help you stay accountable and motivated.

3. **Integrate Activity Into Daily Life:**

- o **Active Choices:** Look for opportunities to be active throughout your day. Take the stairs instead of the elevator, walk or bike to work, or engage in active hobbies.
- o **Break Up Sedentary Time:** If you have a sedentary job or lifestyle, take regular breaks to stand up, stretch, or move around.

**Mindful Eating Practices for Long-Term Success**

1. **Eat with Intention:**

   - o **Mindful Eating Techniques:** Practice mindful eating by paying full attention to your meals. Focus on the taste, texture, and aroma of your food, and savor each bite.
   - o **Avoid Distractions:** Eat away from distractions such as TVs, phones, or computers. This helps you stay present during meals and recognize hunger and fullness cues.

2. **Portion Awareness:**

   - o **Understand Portions:** Learn to recognize appropriate portion sizes for different foods. Use measuring cups or a food scale if needed to help with portion control.
   - o **Serve Smaller Plates:** Use smaller plates and bowls to help control portion sizes and prevent overeating.

3. **Healthy Snacking:**

   - **Choose Nutritious Snacks:** Opt for healthy snacks that are rich in nutrients and fiber. Fresh fruits, vegetables, nuts, and yogurt are great options.
   - **Plan Ahead:** Prepare and portion snacks in advance to avoid reaching for unhealthy options when you're hungry.

4. **Hydration:**

   - **Stay Hydrated:** Drink plenty of water throughout the day. Adequate hydration supports overall health and can help manage hunger and cravings.
   - **Limit Sugary Drinks:** Avoid sugary beverages like sodas and fruit juices. Opt for water, herbal teas, or flavored water with fresh fruit slices.

# Conclusion

Maintaining your weight loss involves transitioning to a balanced and sustainable approach to eating and living. By adjusting your meal plan, incorporating healthy habits, and staying active, you can successfully manage your weight in the long term. Embrace a lifestyle that supports your goals and fosters overall well-being for lasting success.

In the next chapter, we'll delve into advanced strategies for optimizing your weight management plan and making the most of your healthy lifestyle. Stay tuned for more insights and practical tips!

# Chapter 7: Frequently Asked Questions (FAQs)

Navigating the journey of weight loss and meal planning often brings up a range of questions. This chapter addresses some of the most common concerns and misconceptions, providing practical advice and insights based on real-world experiences.

## Common Questions About Meal Planning and Weight Loss

### 1. How do I start meal planning for weight loss?

### Answer:

Starting meal planning for weight loss involves several key steps:

1. **Set Clear Goals:** Define your weight loss goals and dietary preferences. Determine how many meals and snacks you need each day and your target caloric intake.

2. **Assess Your Current Diet:** Evaluate your current eating habits to identify areas for improvement. Look for patterns in your food choices and consider any nutritional gaps.

3. **Create a Meal Plan Template:** Develop a meal plan template that includes breakfast, lunch, dinner, and snacks for the week. Ensure your plan includes a variety of foods to meet your nutritional needs and prevent boredom.

4. **Prepare a Shopping List:** Based on your meal plan, create a detailed shopping list of all the ingredients you'll need. This helps streamline grocery shopping and ensures you have everything on hand.

5. **Batch Cook and Prep:** Prepare meals or ingredients in advance to save time during the week. Cook in batches and store portions in the fridge or freezer for easy access.

6. **Monitor and Adjust:** Track your progress and make adjustments to your meal plan as needed. Pay attention to how your body responds and make changes to better align with your goals.

For a comprehensive guide on meal planning, check out this resource from the Academy of Nutrition and Dietetics.

## 2. Can I lose weight without counting calories?

**Answer:**

Yes, it's possible to lose weight without meticulously counting calories by focusing on other strategies:

1. **Portion Control:** Use portion control techniques to manage your food intake. Avoid overeating by serving smaller portions and eating mindfully.

2. **Emphasize Whole Foods:** Prioritize whole, nutrient-dense foods like fruits, vegetables, lean proteins, and whole grains. These foods are generally lower in calories and higher in nutrients.

3. **Listen to Your Body:** Pay attention to hunger and fullness cues. Eat when you're hungry and stop when you're satisfied, rather than eating based on a predetermined calorie limit.

4. **Practice Mindful Eating:** Engage in mindful eating practices to enhance your awareness of what and how much you're eating. This can help prevent overeating and improve your relationship with food.

5. **Focus on Quality Over Quantity:** Choose high-quality foods that nourish your body and support your weight loss goals. Nutrient-dense foods can help you feel fuller longer and reduce overall calorie intake.

Explore this article for more information on losing weight without counting calories.

## 3. How do I handle cravings while on a meal plan?

### Answer:

Managing cravings is a common challenge during a weight loss journey. Here are some strategies to handle cravings effectively:

1. **Identify Triggers:** Understand what triggers your cravings. It might be stress, boredom, or certain environments. By identifying triggers, you can develop strategies to address them.

2. **Healthy Substitutes:** Find healthier alternatives to satisfy your cravings. For example, if you crave sweets, opt for fruit or a small piece of dark chocolate instead of sugary desserts.

3. **Stay Hydrated:** Sometimes cravings are mistaken for thirst. Drink water regularly throughout the day to stay hydrated and curb unnecessary cravings.

4. **Distract Yourself:** Engage in activities that take your mind off cravings. Go for a walk, read a book, or engage in a hobby to shift your focus away from food.

5. **Practice Portion Control:** If you decide to indulge in a craving, do so in moderation. Enjoy a small portion and savor it slowly to prevent

overconsumption.

Learn more about managing cravings in <u>this guide</u> from Medical News Today.

## 4. Is it necessary to exercise to lose weight?

### Answer:

While diet plays a significant role in weight loss, incorporating exercise into your routine can enhance your results and contribute to overall health:

1. **Boosts Calorie Burn:** Exercise increases your calorie expenditure, which can help create a calorie deficit and support weight loss. Both cardiovascular and strength training exercises are beneficial.

2. **Build Muscle Mass:** Strength training exercises help build muscle, which can boost your metabolism and improve body composition. Muscle tissue burns more calories at rest compared to fat tissue.

3. **Improves Fitness and Well-Being:** Regular exercise improves cardiovascular health, enhances mood, and reduces stress. It also supports long-term weight management by promoting a healthy lifestyle.

4. **Supports Appetite Regulation:** Exercise can help regulate appetite hormones and reduce cravings. Engaging in physical activity can help you make healthier food choices.

5. **Enhances Weight Loss Efforts:** Combining exercise with a balanced diet provides a holistic approach to weight loss. It can accelerate progress and improve overall fitness.

For tips on incorporating exercise into your routine, check out this resource from the Centers for Disease Control and Prevention (CDC).

## 5. How do I deal with weight loss plateaus?

### Answer:

Weight loss plateaus are common and can be frustrating. Here's how to deal with them effectively:

1. **Reassess Your Caloric Intake:** As you lose weight, your caloric needs change. Recalculate your daily caloric requirements and adjust your intake accordingly to continue progressing.

2. **Modify Your Exercise Routine:** Introduce variety into your exercise routine to challenge your body in new ways. Increase intensity, try new workouts, or incorporate interval training.

3. **Check for Non-Scale Victories:** Look for progress beyond the scale, such as improvements in fitness, energy levels, or clothing fit. These indicators can provide motivation and show that you're making progress.

4. **Evaluate Your Meal Plan:** Review your meal plan to ensure it aligns with your current goals and needs. Make adjustments to portion sizes, food choices, or meal frequency if necessary.

5. **Stay Consistent and Patient:** Plateaus are a normal part of the weight loss process. Stay consistent with your efforts and be patient. Trust the process and make gradual adjustments as needed.

Explore more strategies for overcoming plateaus in this article from Healthline.

## 6. What should I do if I slip up or have an off day?

### Answer:

Experiencing a slip-up or an off day is a natural part of any weight loss journey. Here's how to handle it effectively:

1. **Don't Dwell on It:** Avoid dwelling on a slip-up or feeling guilty. Acknowledge it, learn from it, and

move forward without letting it derail your progress.

2. **Get Back on Track:** Resume your healthy habits as soon as possible. Return to your meal plan and exercise routine to regain momentum.

3. **Analyze What Happened:** Reflect on the circumstances that led to the slip-up. Identify any patterns or triggers and develop strategies to address them in the future.

4. **Practice Self-Compassion:** Be kind to yourself and recognize that weight loss is a journey with ups and downs. Treat yourself with compassion and stay focused on your long-term goals.

5. **Seek Support:** If you're struggling to get back on track, seek support from friends, family, or a weight loss coach. They can provide encouragement and help you stay accountable.

Learn more about dealing with setbacks in this guide from Psychology Today.

## 7. How can I stay motivated during my weight loss journey?

**Answer:**

Maintaining motivation throughout your weight loss journey is crucial for success. Here are some strategies to stay motivated:

1. **Set Achievable Goals:** Set clear, realistic, and achievable goals. Break your long-term goals into smaller milestones and celebrate each achievement.

2. **Track Your Progress:** Keep track of your progress using a journal, app, or photos. Seeing your progress visually can boost motivation and provide a sense of accomplishment.

3. **Create a Support System:** Build a support network of friends, family, or a weight loss group. Share your goals and progress with them for encouragement and accountability.

4. **Stay Inspired:** Find sources of inspiration, such as success stories, motivational quotes, or personal affirmations. Surround yourself with positive influences that reinforce your commitment.

5. **Make It Enjoyable:** Incorporate activities you enjoy into your routine, such as favorite workouts, cooking new recipes, or engaging in hobbies. Making your journey enjoyable can help maintain motivation.

Explore more tips for staying motivated in <u>this article</u> from Verywell Fit.

## 8. Are there any specific foods that can aid weight loss?

## Answer:

Certain foods can support weight loss due to their nutritional properties. Here are some examples:

1. **Lean Proteins:** Foods like chicken breast, turkey, tofu, and fish are high in protein and can help build muscle and keep you full longer.

2. **Fiber-Rich Foods:** Vegetables, fruits, legumes, and whole grains are rich in fiber, which helps keep you full and supports digestive health. Fiber slows digestion and promotes satiety, reducing overall calorie intake.

3. **Healthy Fats:** Avocados, nuts, seeds, and olive oil provide healthy fats that can support metabolism and help you feel satisfied. Incorporating these fats in moderation can aid in weight management without causing weight gain.

4. **Lean Dairy:** Low-fat or non-fat dairy products like Greek yogurt and cottage cheese are high in protein and can aid in muscle maintenance and satiety.

5. **Green Tea:** Rich in antioxidants and catechins, green tea may help boost metabolism and promote fat

oxidation. Drinking green tea regularly can complement your weight loss efforts.

**6. Water-Rich Foods:** Foods with high water content, such as cucumbers, watermelon, and soups, can help with hydration and reduce overall calorie consumption.

**7. Spices:** Certain spices, like cayenne pepper, cinnamon, and ginger, can have thermogenic effects, potentially boosting metabolism and aiding weight loss.

For more information on weight loss-friendly foods, check out this article from Healthline.

## 9. How important is meal timing for weight loss?

### Answer:

Meal timing can impact weight loss and overall health in several ways:

1. **Consistent Meal Times:** Eating at regular intervals can help regulate hunger hormones and prevent overeating. Aim to eat meals and snacks at consistent times each day to maintain balanced energy levels.

2. **Pre-Workout Nutrition:** Eating a small, balanced meal or snack before exercise can provide the energy needed for a productive workout and enhance performance.

3. **Post-Workout Nutrition:** Consuming protein and carbohydrates after exercise helps with muscle recovery and replenishes glycogen stores. This can support continued weight loss and muscle maintenance.

4. **Avoid Late-Night Eating:** Eating large meals late at night may disrupt sleep and lead to weight gain. Aim to finish eating at least 2-3 hours before bedtime.

5. **Intermittent Fasting:** Some people find intermittent fasting beneficial for weight loss. This approach involves cycling between periods of eating and fasting. However, it's important to choose a method that suits your lifestyle and preferences.

Learn more about meal timing and its impact on weight loss in this guide from Medical News Today.

**10. Can I lose weight with a vegetarian or vegan diet?**

**Answer:**

Yes, it's possible to lose weight with a vegetarian or vegan diet. Here's how to do it effectively:

1. **Plan Balanced Meals:** Ensure your vegetarian or vegan diet includes a variety of nutrient-dense foods, such as fruits, vegetables, legumes, whole

grains, nuts, and seeds. This helps provide essential nutrients and prevent deficiencies.

2. **Monitor Protein Intake:** Include plant-based protein sources like beans, lentils, tofu, tempeh, and quinoa to meet your protein needs. Adequate protein is important for muscle maintenance and satiety.

3. **Watch for Hidden Calories:** Be mindful of high-calorie plant-based foods like nuts, avocados, and plant-based cheeses. While these foods are healthy, portion control is key to managing calorie intake.

4. **Focus on Whole Foods:** Prioritize whole, minimally processed foods over processed vegetarian or vegan products, which may be high in sugars, fats, and calories.

5. **Supplement Wisely:** Consider supplements for nutrients that may be harder to obtain from a plant-based diet, such as vitamin B12, vitamin D, omega-3 fatty acids, and iron.

Explore more about weight loss on a vegetarian or vegan diet in this article from the Academy of Nutrition and Dietetics.

# 11. What should I do if I have a medical condition affecting my weight?

## Answer:

If you have a medical condition that affects your weight, it's important to approach weight management with special considerations:

1. **Consult a Healthcare Provider:** Work with your healthcare provider to develop a personalized weight management plan. They can help address any underlying health issues and recommend appropriate strategies.

2. **Follow Medical Advice:** Adhere to any dietary or lifestyle recommendations provided by your healthcare provider. They may suggest specific dietary modifications or medications to support your weight management.

3. **Monitor Symptoms:** Keep track of how your weight management efforts affect your condition. If you experience any changes in symptoms or new concerns, communicate with your healthcare provider promptly.

4. **Work with a Dietitian:** A registered dietitian can help you create a meal plan tailored to your medical condition and nutritional needs. They can provide guidance on managing your condition while

working towards your weight loss goals.

5. **Seek Support:** Consider joining a support group or working with a counselor to address any emotional or psychological aspects related to managing your condition and weight.

For more information on managing weight with medical conditions, refer to this guide from WebMD.

## 12. How can I make meal planning more enjoyable?

### Answer:

Making meal planning enjoyable can help you stay motivated and engaged in your weight loss journey. Here are some tips:

1. **Get Creative:** Experiment with new recipes and ingredients to keep your meals exciting. Try cooking classes, food blogs, or culinary apps for inspiration.

2. **Involve Family and Friends:** Involve family or friends in meal planning and preparation. Cooking together can make the process more fun and provide additional support.

3. **Use Meal Planning Apps:** Utilize meal planning apps or websites to streamline the process. Many apps offer customizable meal plans, recipes, and

shopping lists to make planning easier.

4. **Make it a Ritual:** Set aside a specific time each week for meal planning. Turn it into a relaxing ritual by listening to music or enjoying a favorite beverage while you plan.

5. **Celebrate Your Successes:** Reward yourself for sticking to your meal plan and achieving milestones. Celebrate with a healthy treat, a fun activity, or a relaxing break.

Explore meal planning tools and resources in <u>this guide</u> from BBC Good Food.

# Conclusion

Addressing these frequently asked questions can help clarify common concerns and misconceptions about meal planning and weight loss. By understanding and applying these insights, you can enhance your weight loss journey and create a more sustainable and enjoyable approach to meal planning. If you have additional questions or need further guidance, don't hesitate to seek support from professionals or resources tailored to your specific needs.

In the next chapter, we will provide additional tips and advanced strategies for optimizing your meal planning and weight loss efforts. Stay tuned for more practical advice and expert insights!

# Chapter 8: Conclusion

## Final Thoughts

As we reach the end of this journey together, it's important to take a moment to reflect on the key takeaways from this eBook and to consider how you can apply these insights to achieve your weight loss goals. This eBook has been designed to provide you with practical, actionable advice and strategies for creating healthy meal plans that support effective and sustainable weight loss. Let's recap the main points covered:

### 1. Understanding Your Weight Loss Goals

Setting realistic weight loss goals is essential for success. By determining your ideal weight and caloric needs, and tracking your progress, you can stay focused and motivated throughout your journey. Remember to set achievable targets and regularly monitor your progress to stay on track.

### 2. The Foundations of a Healthy Diet

A healthy diet is built on understanding macronutrients and micronutrients. By balancing proteins, carbohydrates, and fats, and ensuring adequate intake of essential vitamins and minerals, you can create a diet that supports weight loss and overall health. Hydration is also a crucial component, as adequate water intake supports metabolism and helps manage hunger.

## 3. Creating Your Weight Loss Meal Plan

Building a balanced plate involves understanding portion sizes and food groups to create meals that are both satisfying and conducive to weight loss. Effective meal planning includes preparing meals ahead of time and customizing plans based on your preferences and dietary needs. The sample 7-day meal plan provided in this eBook offers a practical framework to help you get started.

## 4. Adapting Meal Plans to Your Lifestyle

Life can be busy, and adapting meal plans to fit your schedule is crucial for success. Meal prep techniques, quick recipes, and strategies for eating out and handling social situations will help you stay on track even when life gets hectic.

## 5. Overcoming Common Weight Loss Challenges

Challenges such as cravings, emotional eating, and weight loss plateaus are common. This chapter provided techniques for managing cravings, breaking through plateaus, and staying motivated throughout your weight loss journey. Addressing these challenges head-on will help you maintain your progress and continue moving towards your goals.

## 6. Long-Term Weight Management

Transitioning to maintenance after achieving your weight loss goals requires adjustments to your meal plan and lifestyle. Incorporating healthy habits, such as regular exercise and mindful eating practices, will help you sustain your weight loss and continue leading a healthy lifestyle.

## 7. Frequently Asked Questions (FAQs)

Understanding common questions and concerns about meal planning and weight loss can provide clarity and practical solutions to common issues. From handling slip-ups to managing weight with medical conditions, the FAQs chapter aimed to address real-world experiences and offer valuable advice.

## Encouragement to Start Implementing the Meal Plans and Tips Provided

Now that you have a comprehensive understanding of how to create effective meal plans for weight loss, it's time to put these strategies into action. Implementing the meal plans and tips provided in this eBook will set you on the path to achieving your weight loss goals. Remember that the journey may have its ups and downs, but consistency and commitment are key to success.

Start by:

1. **Setting Up Your Meal Plan:** Use the sample meal plans as a template and customize them according to your preferences and nutritional needs. Begin with a week of planned meals and adjust as

necessary.

2. **Prepping Your Meals:** Implement meal prep techniques to save time and ensure you have healthy options readily available. This will make it easier to stick to your plan and avoid unhealthy choices.

3. **Tracking Your Progress:** Regularly monitor your progress, including any changes in weight, energy levels, and overall well-being. Use this information to make adjustments to your meal plan and stay motivated.

4. **Staying Flexible:** Life is unpredictable, so be prepared to adapt your meal plan as needed. If you encounter obstacles or setbacks, adjust your approach and continue moving forward.

5. **Seeking Support:** Don't hesitate to reach out for support or guidance if needed. Whether it's connecting with a dietitian, joining a support group, or engaging with online communities, seeking help can enhance your weight loss journey.

## Call to Action

I invite you to connect with me on social media or through my website for additional support and resources. Engaging with a community of like-minded individuals can provide motivation, inspiration, and accountability. Stay updated with the latest tips, recipes, and advice by following my social media channels or visiting my website.

- **Follow me on Instagram for daily tips and motivation.**
- **Join our Facebook group to connect with others on their weight loss journey.**
- **Visit my website for more resources, articles, and personalized support.**

Your commitment to making positive changes is commendable, and I am here to support you every step of the way. Together, we can achieve your weight loss goals and build a healthier, more fulfilling life.

Thank you for joining me on this journey. I wish you success and happiness in achieving your weight loss and wellness goals!

# Chapter 9: Appendices

## Appendix A: Grocery Shopping List

To make your weight loss journey easier, here's a comprehensive grocery shopping list based on the meal plans provided in this eBook. This list includes a variety of ingredients needed to prepare healthy and delicious meals. You can use this as a reference to ensure you have everything you need for your weekly meal prep.

# Produce:

- **Fruits:**

    - Apples
    - Bananas
    - Berries (strawberries, blueberries, raspberries)
    - Oranges
    - Grapes
    - Lemons
    - Avocados
    - Watermelon
    - Tomatoes
- **Vegetables:**

    - Spinach

- o Kale
- o Broccoli
- o Cauliflower
- o Bell peppers (red, yellow, green)
- o Carrots
- o Cucumbers
- o Zucchini
- o Sweet potatoes
- o Onions
- o Garlic
- o Mushrooms
- **Herbs:**

  - o Fresh parsley
  - o Fresh basil
  - o Fresh cilantro

## Proteins:

- **Meat and Poultry:**

  - o Chicken breast
  - o Ground turkey
- **Seafood:**

  - o Salmon
  - o Shrimp
- **Plant-Based Proteins:**

  - o Tofu
  - o Tempeh

- o Canned beans (black beans, chickpeas, kidney beans)
  - o Lentils
- **Dairy and Alternatives:**

  - o Greek yogurt (plain, non-fat)
  - o Cottage cheese (low-fat)
  - o Almond milk (unsweetened)

## Grains and Legumes:

- **Whole Grains:**

  - o Quinoa
  - o Brown rice
  - o Oats
- **Legumes:**

  - o Chickpeas
  - o Black beans
  - o Lentils

## Nuts and Seeds:

- Almonds
- Walnuts
- Chia seeds
- Flaxseeds

## Oils and Condiments:

- Olive oil

- Coconut oil
- Apple cider vinegar
- Soy sauce (low sodium)
- Dijon mustard

### Spices and Seasonings:

- Salt (preferably sea salt or Himalayan salt)
- Black pepper
- Paprika
- Cumin
- Turmeric
- Cinnamon
- Chili powder

### Miscellaneous:

- Low-sodium vegetable broth
- Whole grain or sprouted bread
- Nut butter (peanut or almond)

This list can be adjusted based on personal preferences and dietary needs. For an interactive shopping list and meal planning tools, consider using this grocery list app to keep track of your ingredients.

## Appendix B: Meal Plan Templates

To help you create and customize your own meal plans, here are blank templates that you can use. These templates are designed to make meal planning easier and more organized. Simply fill in the meal options and snacks for each day of the week.

## Weekly Meal Plan Template:

# Day 1:

- **Breakfast:**
- **Lunch:**
- **Dinner:**
- **Snacks:**

# Day 2:

- **Breakfast:**
- **Lunch:**
- **Dinner:**
- **Snacks:**

# Day 3:

- **Breakfast:**
- **Lunch:**
- **Dinner:**
- **Snacks:**

# Day 4:

- **Breakfast:**
- **Lunch:**
- **Dinner:**
- **Snacks:**

# Day 5:

- **Breakfast:**
- **Lunch:**
- **Dinner:**
- **Snacks:**

# Day 6:

- **Breakfast:**
- **Lunch:**
- **Dinner:**
- **Snacks:**

# Day 7:

- **Breakfast:**
- **Lunch:**
- **Dinner:**
- **Snacks:**

For printable templates and meal planning tools, visit this meal planning resource.

# Appendix C: Additional Resources

To further support your weight loss journey and provide you with additional tools, here are some recommended books, websites, and apps. These resources offer valuable information, tips, and tools to help you stay on track and achieve your goals.

**Recommended Books:**

- **"The Whole30: The 30-Day Guide to Total Health and Food Freedom"** by Melissa Hartwig Urban and Dallas Hartwig. This book provides a comprehensive guide to resetting your eating habits and achieving better health through a 30-day elimination diet.

  - Read More
- **"Intuitive Eating: A Revolutionary Program That Works"** by Evelyn Tribole and Elyse Resch. This book offers insights into listening to your body's hunger cues and developing a healthier relationship with food.

  - Read More
- **"The Obesity Code: Unlocking the Secrets of Weight Loss"** by Dr. Jason Fung. This book explores the science behind obesity and provides strategies for managing weight through diet and lifestyle changes.

- o [Read More](#)

## Recommended Websites:

- **Healthline**: Offers a wide range of articles and resources on nutrition, weight loss, and healthy living.
- **Eat Right**: Provides evidence-based information on diet and nutrition from the Academy of Nutrition and Dietetics.
- **MyFitnessPal**: A popular app and website for tracking food intake, exercise, and progress towards weight loss goals.

## Recommended Apps:

- **MyFitnessPal**: A comprehensive app for tracking calories, exercise, and nutritional information.
- **Yummly**: Offers personalized recipe recommendations and meal planning tools.
- **SparkPeople**: Provides a range of resources for meal planning, fitness tracking, and community support.

These additional resources are designed to provide ongoing support and information as you continue on your weight loss journey. Whether you're seeking new recipes, tracking tools, or expert advice, these books, websites, and apps can be valuable assets in your efforts to achieve and maintain your health and weight goals.

www.ingramcontent.com/pod-product-compliance
Lightning Source LLC
Chambersburg PA
CBHW081439250726
48662CB00009B/2860